The ON

C000146077

In a Nutshell

Georges Philips & Simon Shawcross

Published by Copeland and Wickson

The ONE Diet — In a Nutshell

First published 2012

ISBN-13: 978-1904928041
ISBN-10: 1-904928048

www.theonediet.com

Prologue

This version of *The ONE Diet* is designed to give you a broad perspective of the philosophy and methodology that underpins our approach to weight loss.

We have selected sections from the original book that we feel will be most useful to you. Included are the powerfully concise *In a nutshell* and *In conclusion* segments, as well as elements of psychology, nutrition and fitness that we believe will help give sufficient information to enable you to benefit.

The research and in depth detail has been omitted here for the sake of brevity and is available to those who want a deeper understanding in the original version. The original book includes recipes, meal suggestions, a full step-by-step guide, more detailed psychology and a comprehensive explanation of food types and the effects they have on us.

We hope that *The ONE Diet – In a Nutshell* will empower you to reach your goals and fulfil your aspirations.

Please feel free to contact us through our website and follow our blog posts. You will find the details in the *Resources* section at the back of the book.

Enjoy the journey.

Georges Philips and Simon Shawcross.

Foreword

The ONE Diet is a perfect name for the book you are about to read. It is not just another in a long string of diets that you have tried…it is THE diet that correlates with the genome within your body that has been evolving over billions of years.

Go get a new roll of toilet paper. Look at it. Let this entire roll represent the history of the human species. Holding the roll in your left hand, tear off a single square of the tissue and hold it in your right hand. What you hold in your left hand represents the amount of time that our species lived off the land as hunter-gatherers. What you hold in your right hand represents the agricultural revolution.

Now, take the square that you hold in your right hand and use a razor blade to cut off the tiniest sliver from the end that you can manage. This tiny sliver represents the twentieth and twenty-first centuries. This is the slice of time where you will live out your life. Within this slice is a growing epidemic of obesity, diabetes, hypertension, heart disease, and depression. Also within this slice is every diet book that has tried to address this problem, using various manipulations of foodstuffs from the agricultural revolution.

Now let us return to the roll of tissue that you are holding in your left hand. Over this entire span of time, there was not a single obese human. Humans like every other animal, autoregulated to an ideal body composition without even thinking about it. Along with the lack of obesity, anthropologic evidence suggests that the diseases that track along with obesity (diabetes, hypertension, heart disease, etc.) were also not present. Throughout this expanse of time free of obesity and disease, there was just ONE diet. The ONE diet was a hunter-gatherer diet.

The ONE Diet will take you on a journey that begins at the ending. In order to make room in your mind for what the diet that shaped your genome looks like, the authors first must do some house cleaning. My dear friend and co-author John Little is also the authorized biographer of Bruce Lee. I remember watching a video interview of Bruce Lee with John when he was discussing how best to teach a pupil. He likened the learning process to a tea ceremony. Both participants in the tea ceremony have tea in their cups. In order for a teacher to give a pupil his tea, the pupil must be willing to pour his tea out of his cup.

Mr. Philips and Mr. Shawcross also realize the importance of this concept and will painstakingly show you what is wrong with the contemporary Western diet and how it foils your attempts to achieve a healthy body composition. They will show you how and why you have been frustrated. More importantly, they will show how your frustration has been used by marketers and scam artists to manipulate you and get your money.

Having dispelled the "conventional wisdom" that has grown out of the experience within that tiny sliver of time in your right hand, *The ONE Diet* will end at the beginning. The authors will explain what the diet that drove the development of your genome looked like. Once they show you what that diet looked like, they will show how to approximate it in the modern environment. Rather than simply suggesting "Paleo re-enactment," the authors will show you what to avoid in the modern environment and what to include so that the correct metabolic and hormonal environment exists.

One of my favorite aspects of this book is that it focuses on an aspect of body recomposition that all the other books in the Paleo genre have largely ignored: the psychological aspect. The authors understand that no matter how powerful the arguments, or how deep your understanding, if you have unresolved psychological issues you are doomed to failure. Throughout *The ONE Diet*, there are discussions of the potential psychological roadblocks and strategies for how to overcome them.

One of my major dissatisfactions with other books advocating an evolutionary-based diet is that after giving a beautiful treatise shattering the conventional wisdom on diet, they would launch into a discussion of exercise that involved a conventional wisdom that was as inaccurate as the diet they just debunked. Not so with *The ONE Diet*. The authors correctly recommend a high intensity program that is brief and infrequent. Such an approach to exercise creates an optimal metabolic and hormonal environment that will work synergistically with your new diet without creating overtraining or burnout. And rather than trying to cover the exercise topic as extensively as the diet, they simply outline a solid starting point and make appropriate references for readers who want more.

You now hold in your hands *The ONE Diet*. It is NOT the next new thing. It is a very old thing...billions of years in the making. It is what drove the evolution of the genome which makes up your body. It cannot fail. As the philosopher, Francis Bacon said: "Nature, to be commanded, must be obeyed."
In Health and Strength,

M. Doug McGuff, MD
Co-Author of *Body by Science*

Introduction

"My health is the main capital I have and I want to administer it intelligently."

Ernest Hemingway

The weight loss obsession seems to be sweeping the developed nations at a phenomenal rate.

No matter where you are, there appear reminders that we are the wrong size, that someone's ice cream is much tastier, and that we can look years younger with this special cream. There is a pandemic all about size and appearance.

Yet here we are on the treadmill of life, as far as our size is concerned, experiencing frustration, discomfort, disease, and even feeling guilty for being unable to reach that elusive "right size," instead heading more toward "supersize."

Generally, people do not plan to fail. They do not set out deliberately to make something more difficult than it need be. They certainly do not throw money away unnecessarily on a hopeless idea, some miracle potion or magical gadget.

Most people are well intentioned and honorable. Often they are following a formula they believe will get them to be the right shape and size, to no avail. However, if you were playing a sport whose rules you did not fully understand, would you not agree that the chances of success are going to be minimal and that you are likely to consistently lose?

Weight loss rules are simple, though for most people, not yet transparent. This means that unless you have a full understanding of the mechanism that determines what shape and size you can best be and the rules that need to be followed, you are likely to fail. Success comes to those who have both an understanding and the determination to make it happen.

We believe that for most readers, this is unlikely to be the first weight loss book invested in. In other words, most readers are determined to find a solution. What has been lacking for most in the past is not determination; rather, it has been the understanding.

It is not that people plan to fail, rather that they simply fail to plan. Weight loss, perhaps, attracts more than its fair share of those people. It is not that they are not capable; rather, they start with the premise that losing weight is going to be easy and they will miraculously reach their size and weight goals effortlessly.

Little attention, if any, is given to the reality of weight loss. It is not their fault, nor have they invited the degree of deception that exists in the weight loss industry. Most people have been suckered and hoodwinked by an industry that, in many cases, is ignorant at best and often deliberately misleading.

It is as though the blind are leading the blind. The situation has become so out of control that for most people, weight loss has become a lifelong struggle that seems to keep many at best confused, and at worst miserably depressed.

This book is about the journey required to finally be in control of our weight and size. It is a book about a change of perception through sound nutritional research and a better understanding of human behavior.

The ONE Diet is a reality check. It goes a long way toward shattering illusions that have become embedded in our psyche. A ship, over time, collects barnacles that attach beneath the surface of the water, slowing the flow and distorting the direction, and the vessel needs to be brought to dry dock and serviced. So too we need to stop and examine the misconceptions that we have picked up over time.

In order to create physical change, we need to change our mental attitudes and understanding of what is required to achieve success. In order to do this, we need to challenge the basis on which we have built our misconceptions.

The ONE Diet is as much to do with mind-sets and attitudes as it is about nutrition and diet. It is all encompassing, in the sense that it covers the physiology and the psychology of weight control.

In order to get to grips with weight and size issues, we need to examine all of the relevant aspects involved—this includes the way foods are being sold to us. We explore the degree of persuasion we are open to and how the food industry utilizes our "blind spots" to capitalize on sales. This type of pervasive persuasion is perhaps at the core of how it has become so difficult to be free of excess weight.

There is little doubt that reading this book will have an effect. We would go a little further and suggest that "you cannot not be affected" by reading *The ONE Diet – In a Nutshell*. It is simply because the evidence is so overwhelming that a change in attitude towards weight is a given.

In order to get the maximum from reading the material, we would suggest that you set some time aside to invest in your self-betterment. It will require that you suspend your disbelief about some things not being good for you when in fact they are and accept that ultimately, what happens to your size is what you decide will happen.

In order to succeed at weight loss, we need to understand how it has become the way it is. We need to understand the assumptions we are making and acquire new knowledge. We need to make informed decisions about what to eat and how to start with a plan that we know will have positive effects. We need to review our relationship with and outlook toward food, to re-establish ourselves as masters of our destiny. *The ONE Diet – In a Nutshell* is a road map to your successful weight loss program.

Chapter 1.

The Miracle Industry

IN A NUTSHELL:

- There are many gimmicky products, books, and services out there looking to capture a portion of the weight loss market. Be aware that you don't fall prey to their outlandish claims. The weight loss industry is now worth between $33 billion and $55 billion per year in the United States alone.

- In the West, we are often held to ransom between a food industry that continually supplies an overabundance of the wrong foods and a miracle weight loss industry promising to solve our weight issues "overnight." No product or service can better a natural, healthy diet that you adhere to over the long term.

- Models used in advertising to promote unhealthy foods are never overweight; they always appear slim, happy, and smiling. Modeling is a profession; they are paid well to remain in good shape, stay lean, and smile.

- Almost any diet approach may appear effective in the first four weeks or so due to the body's release of excess water and recovery from systemic inflammation.

- Water loss can account for two to ten pounds per week of weight lost in the first few weeks of a diet, and many popular diets rely on this to appear effective.

- If you are truly prepared to do what is required to healthily lose weight and keep it off, all the information you need is contained within The ONE Diet.

IN CONCLUSION:

- Stay focused and alert to the various marketing methods used to attract your attention to "miracle cures."

- In the old days, "miracle snake oil" salesmen were chased out of town or worse. Regrettably, that is no longer legal. The best we can do is not give any of our precious attention to such hogwash.

- Stay as pure to your needs as your purse allows. Through your actions, you can teach your world that you are not prepared to accept kaka foods, nor will you support the growth of an industry that puts profit before people.

- Very low-calorie diets are usually a problematic approach to weight loss, often resulting in increased weight gain in the long term.

- The ONE Diet will enable you to achieve your ideal weight naturally.

Chapter 2.

Food in the Modern World

IN A NUTSHELL:

- The weight gain and obesity epidemic is a result of unhealthy, over-processed, sweetened, refined, and fake foods. Most of us who want to lose weight are caught up between the mass food industry and the miracle weight loss industry—a vicious cycle.

- Food advertising has become very sophisticated, and advertisers now know how to press our "want it now" buttons. In many instances, we are misled and left confused by both governments and the food industry, which both have vested interests.

- We live in a world where experts in the field of human behavioral persuasion are engaged in applying their skills to change our eating habits for the sole benefit of their companies.

- In the mass food market, although there appear to be ever-increasing numbers of different products, in reality our choices are becoming more limited. Recall the "any customer can have a car painted any color that he wants as long as it is black" principle, made famous by Henry Ford.

IN CONCLUSION:

- No person, organization, corporation, or government can be relied on to have our best interests at heart. It is up to us to champion our self-interest and challenge all information presented to us.

- Conflicting messages and the use of disinformation and corporate spin have infiltrated and infected our notion of eating well.

- By having the right information, we can make better choices and avoid being stuck in a web of deception. Consuming real food and avoiding processed products will improve the quality of our lives and make our weight loss goals obtainable.

- Challenging our own beliefs, our habitual shopping behavior, as well the information presented to us is now vital if we are to be free of the illusions.

Chapter 3.

What's Really Going Wrong

IN A NUTSHELL:

- Carbohydrates are sugars and starches (starches are the more complex sugars).

- The problem of obesity and weight gain in today's world lies in the dramatic increase in the consumption of calories derived from refined carbohydrates (primarily from grains, sugars, and sweeteners).

- Grains, including whole grains, cause additional distress to the human metabolism due to their antinutrient content (gluten is one example of a grain antinutrient).

- Modern chemically altered sweeteners, like high fructose corn syrup, that are major ingredients in many processed foods and drinks substantially compound the weight gain problem.

- The vast majority of the food industry focuses on maximizing profit by selling us cheap-to-produce "foods" and "drinks" loaded with refined carbohydrates. These processed foods are far removed from being "real foods."

- Low-quality and processed foods can stimulate increased hunger and, in some cases, may send us into an eating frenzy. Refined carbohydrates for instance can have similar physiological, addictive effects to recreational drugs.

IN CONCLUSION:

- Stopping the consumption of cereal grains and refined carbohydrates helps to turn the body from fat-storage to fat-burning mode.

- To reduce body fat, most people need to consume fewer than 100 grams of carbohydrates a day, and the carbohydrates we do eat need to come from vegetables and fruit in our diet.

- Watch out for foods that are sold as "healthy" but actually contain grains and/or other unhealthy ingredients, and avoid artificial low-calorie sweeteners.

- Initially, when reducing carbohydrates, be prepared for short-term withdrawal symptoms. Break the sugar addiction and expect to lose around one to two pounds or 0.5 to one kilogram of body fat per week.

- Within a few weeks, your desire for sweet foods will naturally fade away.

- The original human diet as outlined in *The ONE Diet – In a Nutshell* is the antidote, a diet based on animal proteins and fats, vegetables and fruits.

Chapter 4.

The Power of Fats and Proteins

IN A NUTSHELL:

- In recent history, many healthy fats have been maligned by bad science, government agencies, the food industry, and the mass media.

- Saturated fats are in fact a great source of energy for our hearts and bodies. They are rich in energy and improve the functioning of the lungs, kidneys, our immune system, and cell membranes. Eating both fat and protein helps to decrease hunger and control appetite.

- Saturated fat is rich in valuable vitamins, notably A, D and K2, which aid the absorption of important minerals in our diet.

- We also need a balance of omega-3 and omega-6 polyunsaturated fats. Most of us in the West get far too much omega-6, which is found in vegetable, grain and seed oils. Omega-6 has the effect of thickening the blood, whereas omega-3 (found in oily fish, meat and eggs) thins the blood, reduces inflammation, and helps repair the body.

- Modern fats are not healthy for us; these include hydrogenated/partially hydrogenated fat, trans fats, interesterified fats (essentially a new type of trans fat), and fats/oils derived from vegetables, grains and seeds (the two exceptions to this rule are coconut oil and olive oil which are acceptable).

- Fat-free, low-fat, and reduced-fat processed foods and drinks are unnatural and are more likely to cause weight gain.

- Protein is vital for our health and weight loss goals. By far the best sources of protein are meat, game, eggs, fish and poultry.

- Legumes and pulses (mature beans and peas, including soybeans, lentils and peanuts) are poor sources of protein. They are usually best minimized in our diet.

IN CONCLUSION:

- By consuming natural fats like full fat butter, ghee, lard, cheese, eggs, animal fats, and coconut oil, and avoiding vegetable, grain, and seed oils, margarines, hydrogenated/partially hydrogenated fats, and trans fats, we revert to eating as nature intended.

- For optimal health, we need to consume both saturated fats and unsaturated fats as provided by The ONE Diet.

- Avoid all processed foods that are marketed as fat-free, low-fat, or reduced-fat.

- Whenever you can, purchase meat and eggs from animals that have been raised on pasture rather than grain, as they contain increased omega-3 content.

- Avoid modern/Western soy products like fake "meat" and soy protein powders.

Chapter 5.

Our Minds May Make Us Fat

IN A NUTSHELL:

- The mindset, perspective, and attitude we adopt affect our experience and our reactions. The way we communicate with others and, more importantly, with ourselves can have a massive impact on our life experience.

- Our psychology requires close examination if we are to avoid being trapped by historical continuity. The tendency is to continue doing what we have always done, what's known, and what we have become accustomed to.

- Many are trapped by past traumas and events, such as childhood bullying, which result in weight gain. Boredom and loneliness can also result in some of us eating excessively just to fill time and distract us from pain.

- Some of us may have developed "Why should I do what they tell me" or "I don't care" attitudes, even if they are not in our best interests. This type of self-destructive behavior and self-sabotage can lead to serious long-term damage.

- The internal dialogue (how and what we say to ourselves) and our spoken words impact on our actions—be aware of what you are saying to yourself and others.

- Seeking to fit in and be part of a group often results in adopting attitudes and habits that are contrary to our best interest. The cost of "fitting in" can have a very high price tag. Additionally, it can also elevate our stress levels and, consequently, negatively impact our lives.

- In essence, though, it is our beliefs that determine what we experience in our lives. Our beliefs (programming) about our self-image perpetuate our shape and size. These programs have been instilled by others and adopted by us as if they are true. Few challenge the origins of beliefs born in childhood.

- We are driven by our emotions. These tend to be the pursuit of pleasure or the avoidance of pain. Pain is mostly evidenced as fear, whereas pleasure is evidenced as joy. By becoming, aware of our current habits surrounding food, nutrition, and eating, we can ensure we are serving our goals; otherwise, they will need to be constructively changed.

- The tendency is to experience emotions before our mind has had a chance to think through a situation. Once an emotion has been felt, we are blinded to other possibilities. This results in our forgoing the need to think something through and explore other perspectives.

- Some of us may have developed obsessive behaviors, addictions, and compulsions around food. These will need to be addressed. In some cases, seeking professional help may be beneficial.

IN CONCLUSION:

- Be aware of the relationship you have with food and eating—watch out for psychological triggers that may cause you to overeat unhealthy foods. Explore your presuppositions and challenge where they no longer serve your best interest.

- Our mind is averse to change and will do what it can to maintain its present course. Only you can make change happen. Remember that you can't make change happen by just saying what you are going to do. Change happens only when you make it happen in reality.

- Be aware of your habits and compulsions relating to food.

Chapter 6.

Your Best Body Within

IN A NUTSHELL:

- Waking up to the reality of their current size and weight can be a shock for some people. For some, this shock spurs them into action; for others, they manage to bury the reality and carry on as usual.

- Some give up on their goal of losing weight because they've had unsuccessful attempts in the past using very low-calorie diets or complex, convoluted diet systems.

- Successful weight loss will require an initial investment in terms of time, planning, and determination. We will need to be focused and set realistic goals. Weight loss takes time and patience.

- Be aware that some of the people in your life may not want to see you successfully change and may even look to sabotage your progress. Also, be aware of self-sabotage, where those little "nibbles" and "treats" may undermine your progress; keep a daily food diary initially.

- Avoid comparing yourself with others; focus on your own progress and actualizing your best shape. Observe your beliefs about your size, weight, shape, and eating habits, and challenge these where necessary.

- There are certain varying body type characteristics and genes that control, to a degree, how lean an individual can be. This is a reason that comparing yourself with others is usually unproductive and often frustrating.

- No matter what your current size, eating healthily over the long term will optimize your body shape. You will become the best physical version of yourself that you can be. Being in the best shape you can be has many advantages, including being able to look after yourself well into your golden years.

IN CONCLUSION:

- Base your expectations in reality. Set yourself realistic goals—aim for one to two pounds or 0.5 to one kilogram of fat loss per week. There is no need and no point in making comparisons with others; instead, keep track of your physical condition and chart your progress caringly.

- Look out for those people who seek to demoralize and disempower you. They may come appearing to care whilst in reality they have a hidden agenda. Avoid the blame game and accept that you and only you are in control of what you put in your mouth.

- Where no goal has been set, the mind will keep doing what it has always done, by default. Setting and keeping a goal in mind instructs the mind as to where you are heading. Keep focused, keep realistic expectations, and relentlessly maintain your desire for a healthier shape and size.

- Planning, determination, and timing are important aspects of successful weight loss.

Chapter 7.

Excess Fat — What Winners Lose

IN A NUTSHELL:

- Weighing scales don't tell the full picture — we won't know whether weight lost or gained comes from water, muscle, or fat. Obsessive weighing can undermine our good intentions.

- If the scale shows no weight loss, we may get angry. Yet our weight may have stayed the same due to an increase in muscle tissue at the same time as fat loss. The constant use of weighing scales only erodes your personal power and suggests doubt in your abilities to accomplish your goal.

- If you are going to use scales, only do so once a week, at the same time, on the same day. If one week's readings don't show improvement, stay calm — only if a trend happens for two or three weeks in a row will you need to reassess your diet.

- Fluid retention can fluctuate by as much as five pounds or two kilograms in a single day for some people. This is true particularly for women during their monthly cycle.

- If you slip up on your diet or have a "cheat" day, don't be surprised if your scale weight jumps up. Most of this increase will be water rather than fat—so long as it is only a short-term slip up. Obviously fat will accumulate again if you continually eat poorly.

IN CONCLUSION:

- Think of long-term trends, not short-term readings— losing fourteen pounds or six kilograms in two months is good going. Even if you lose more scale weight, it is likely you will have only lost around one to two pounds or 0.5 to one kilogram of actual fat in a week. So look at your objective as long term for a long-lasting result.

- By avoiding the constant weighing and measuring, you are in effect increasing your self-belief. You will, through your actions, teach your mind that you are expecting change at the right pace and the right time, based on your new eating regime. There are many hurdles to overcome, so it does not help adding unnecessary and worthless pressure.

Chapter 8.

Powerful Planning for Success

IN A NUTSHELL:

- Plan ahead and decide a realistic weight or size you want to achieve. By learning to balance the dreamer, the pragmatist, and the critic inside yourself, you are likely to experience a newfound determination. It will also help you to establish emotional balance within your mind and body.

- Affirmations and positive self-talk can be beneficial, but they can also be harmful if not structured in a realistic way. Affirmations must contain an element of truth pertinent to you, not just wishful thinking.

- Learn what your personal anchors and triggers are with regard to your eating patterns; focus on altering the negative ones. Anchors are "on the air", on billboards, in shop windows, etc. Be aware that marketers and advertisers are vying for your attention; they will make you plenty of "irresistible" offers. Resist this buy-in loop if the product on offer is not in your best interests.

- For some people a "Just do it!" attitude is essential for success, like a horse with blinkers; their line of vision is focused only on winning the race.

- Avoid judging both yourself and others. Keep in mind that all judgment is self-judgment. What you say of and to others, you also apply to yourself. Focus on your strengths, support yourself, and show genuine care for yourself through this process. By avoiding playing the victim, "poor me," or "it's not fair" games, you will further develop your self-esteem and self-worth.

- Be aware that we can sometimes distort, delete, and generalize information to suit existing patterns in our minds. When we are looking to make changes, we need to ensure clarity in our thinking and understanding.

- Appreciate that of the words we use, some can be damaging to our mind-set and actions. These include "don't," "ought," "should," "must," "but," "try," "wish," and "hope." Also learn to say, "Thank you…no," when loved ones and friends suggest eating something or offer a gift of something you know will undo your weight loss.

- You will need to choose to change some of your nutritional habits if you are going to attain the goal of weight loss. Confident decisions and actions combined with correct persistence are essential.

IN CONCLUSION:

- Planning ahead for your food shopping and what you will eat tomorrow is empowering yourself and brings greater stability and reduces fear in your mind. Inform your mind through your actions and planning that there will always be quality food available for you.

- Keep your language constructive rather than destructive. Keep it simple by adjusting your responses to "I can," "I need," "I want," and "Thank you...no," as well as "That's not possible" when you have no need. These responses, once mastered, will further direct your mind to your intentions.

- Be vigilant of your mind's distortions by seeking to get all the facts. Be cautious of what your mind deletes, especially concerning your food intake. A food diary can help to minimize the possibility of mentally deleting what you have consumed. Generalizations can excuse and cover up all sorts of misdemeanors, so be aware. Telling yourself, "Well, my friend is on a diet, and she is eating kaka cereal," so as to make it okay for you to eat it, is not clever.

- Focus on extracting all the nutritional information from this book and begin making positive changes to your dietary habits. Become aware of the foods you are buying and eating.

- You always have choice. Exercise your right to choose to eat well; after all, your body may not be the one that you would have designed for yourself yet, but it is not a trash can.

Chapter 9.

The ONE Diet "In a Nutshell"

HOW TO EAT HEALTHILY AND LOSE WEIGHT

The key to eating well and maximizing your weight loss is to combine a protein/fat option (1), with vegetables or salad (2), cooked in and/or dressed with a healthy fat (3), from the **DO EAT** *list on the next page, at every main meal.*

For convenience, you may choose to omit vegetables/salad at breakfast.

It is best to eliminate or at least minimize between-meal snacks. It will serve you best if any snacks you do have consist of an item from the four categories of healthy snacks (4) or a combination, e.g., sliced apple with cheddar cheese. Selecting items from the healthy snack options is also a great way to create a quick and easy breakfast.

Unless noted otherwise, you do not need to limit your consumption of the foods listed in categories 1- 4 of the **DO EAT** *list.*

DO EAT

1. Protein/Fat—Choose from this list: beef, lamb, fish, game, goat, pork, poultry and eggs (if you can, source pastured pork, poultry and eggs as they have a healthier fat profile than the factory reared or grain fed types). Eat between 8–16 ounces (250–500 grams) of animal foods per day.

2. Vegetables/Salad—Almost all vegetables and salad are acceptable and unrestricted. *The only exceptions are:* potatoes, sweet potatoes, yams, parsnips, cassava, and sweet corn. These particular vegetables are potentially too starchy for many people during the process of losing weight. You may experiment with a small portion (equivalent to your fist size or less) of one of these starchy vegetables with a main meal. If your weight loss slows down you will need to further reduce portion size, limit these starchy vegetables to occasional use only, or avoid them altogether whilst it is your goal to lose weight.

3. Healthy Fats—Use these fats for cooking; butter (ideally pastured butter from cows fed grass), lard, ghee and unrefined virgin coconut oil. Use extra virgin olive oil as a salad dressing if you enjoy the flavor. Whole (full-fat) cream or coconut milk can be used in a recipe or a little may be added to a portion of fruit. Ensure it is a pure cream or coconut milk with no added sweeteners/sugars.

4. Healthy Snacks:

a) High quality cured meats, continental sausages, and cold sliced meats that have no added sugars, carbohydrates, or excess chemical preservatives. To be acceptable, a sausage ideally needs to have 90 percent or higher meat content with less than two grams of carbohydrates per sausage or serving. The nutritional information label will show this information.

b) Approved fruits—Limit to one to two portions per day whilst focusing on weight loss. *These fruits are particularly good for us during weight loss:* all varieties of fresh berries, cherries, apples, pears, apricots, peaches, plums, kiwi, pomegranates, figs, prunes, bananas, and grapefruit. *Minimize or, ideally, cut out altogether these fruits whilst reducing your weight, as they have higher sugar content:* grapes, watermelons, melons, dates, mangoes, papayas, pineapples, nectarines, oranges, tangerines, and all dried fruits.

c) Approved nuts—Choose from this list: almonds, walnuts, macadamias, pistachios, hazelnuts, pecans, pine nuts, brazils. If you enjoy the taste of any of these nuts, have an occasional palmful or add them to a salad.

d) Approved cheeses—Mature and hard cheeses (as they contain less lactose (milk sugar) and their protein content is more digestible than soft cheeses) including: cheddar, gorgonzola, parmesan, gouda, edam, emmental and gruyere. Soft cheeses are acceptable if you find they cause you no digestive distress. Avoid processed cheeses altogether.

WHAT TO AVOID

In addition to eating healthy foods from the previous list, it is important for your health and weight loss to avoid the following:

1. **Grains**—Cereal grains, whole grains, refined grains, flours, and products that contain grains—pasta, bread, breakfast cereals, pastries, biscuits, crackers, pies and other bakery goods.

Rice is a partial exception to this rule as it is a nongluten grain and has far fewer inflammatory antinutrients than the gluten grains like wheat. The antinutrient phytin, which is present in the bran of brown rice and wild rice is milled and polished away from the grain during the process used to produce white rice. All remaining antinutrients in white rice are denatured and made safe by exposure to heat (e.g. during cooking). A small portion of white rice may be included as a side to a main meal occasionally during the weight loss process. Unsweetened puffed rice paired with a *small* amount of half-and-half, half cream or whole (full-fat) milk may make a suitable breakfast for some people.

White rice may slow or halt weight loss for some individuals, if this is the case for you, you may need to eliminate rice altogether for a time.

2. **Sugars And Sweeteners**—Foods and drinks that contain added sugars and sweeteners, including table sugar, sucrose, dextrose, fructose, high fructose corn syrup, rice syrup, glucose, artificial sweeteners (saccharine, sucralose, aspartame, etc.), and so on. (These sweeteners are also often present in ready meals, cakes, biscuits, jams, confectionary, desserts, sodas, soft drinks, sports/energy drinks, etc.).

3. **Unhealthy Fats**—Vegetable/grain/seed and nut; oils, fats, and spreads. Hydrogenated oil/fat, partially hydrogenated oil/fat, trans fats, and interesterified fats. Also, avoid products containing these fats; check the nutritional label.

4. **Altered Fat Level Products**—All "low-fat," "fat-free," and "reduced-fat" products. This includes semi-skimmed and skimmed milk, low-fat yoghurts, low-fat cheeses, etc.

5. **Legumes And Pulses**—Soybeans, soya, and all soy products, all mature beans and peas (including dried beans and peas), lentils and peanuts.

Edible immature beans and peas, many of which can be eaten in their pods, are however healthy and perfectly acceptable, including: green beans, french beans, runner beans, string beans, green peas, snap peas, sugarsnap peas, mangetout and snow peas. Treat these immature beans and peas as you would vegetables.

6. **Fruit Juices** — All fruit juices, as they contain far too much sugar.

7. **Junk Food In General** — Ready meals, microwave meals, crisps, chocolate, crackers, fast food/junk food, soft drinks, etc.

8. **Processed Meat** — Sausages and other processed meats that have been filled out with carbohydrates and sugars.

9. **High-Carbohydrate Alcoholic Drinks** — Beer and lager, cider, sweet wines and fortified wines (port, sherry, dessert wines).

By cutting out the items in this list, you will have eliminated the foods and ingredients that are responsible for triggering weight gain. Moreover, you will have taken some of the most beneficial steps possible to improving your long-term health.

ADDITIONAL CONSIDERATIONS

Healthy Ingredients, Sauces, Condiments, Herbs and Spices to Use

Coconut flour

Herbs, fresh if possible (dried if not): coriander, parsley, dill, chives, basil, thyme, rosemary, coriander, etc.

Unrefined organic sea salt

Peppercorns (to grind)

Spices: chili, cumin, paprika, turmeric, cinnamon, garam masala, curry powder, etc.

Ginger

Tomato puree

Vinegars, e.g., balsamic vinegar, white wine vinegar, raw unfiltered cider vinegar

Full-fat homemade mayonnaise (without the vegetable oils used in commercial mayonnaise)

Sour cream

Crème fraiche

Chili sauce

Oyster sauce

Mustards

Dark chocolate (85 percent cocoa or higher)

The Importance Of Hydration

The human body requires water to function, and water does so much for us; it helps keep the body's temperature in equilibrium, it helps our digestive system, and it provides an important function on the cellular level as a lubricator and shock absorber.

Keep yourself well hydrated by drinking approved liquids, throughout the day.

Drinks to Enjoy

Water
Water with a squeeze of fresh orange, lemon, or lime
Coffee
Tea, hot or iced
Herbal teas or iced herbal teas
Cocoa (Dutch-processed cocoa in the United States) made with pure unsweetened cocoa powder (which will ideally have only two listed ingredients: cocoa powder and an acidity regulator like potassium carbonate). Add cream or coconut milk and water to achieve your preferred consistency and taste.

Caffeine Counting

Some older nutritional advice suggests that drinking coffee and tea does not count as water intake as they are diuretics, meaning they can make you excrete water. Coffee and tea are, however, very mild diuretics, and the notion that you will have a net loss of water by drinking them is simply incorrect, unless you consume copious amounts of them. So fret not, because drinking tea and coffee does count as water intake and will hydrate you.

Caffeinated beverages are fine in moderation in a healthy diet. Moderation means up to around 300 grams of caffeine per day. To give you a basis on which to plan your caffeine consumption, here are some typical amounts of caffeine in our approved caffeinated drinks:

Coffee (average cup) — 100 mg

Black tea (average cup) — 50 mg

Green tea (average cup) — 30 mg

White tea (average cup) — 20 mg

Herbal tea — 0 mg

If you have been used to adding sugar or sweeteners to your tea and coffee, you will need to stop doing so. If you absolutely must sweeten your beverages, use raw honey or traditional natural maple syrup (avoid varieties with added sugars or sweeteners, though—check the label!). Be careful to minimize and not go overboard, as they still have a high sugar load. If you can do without, leave them out! We would suggest you work towards cutting even these natural sweeteners out over time anyway *and some people may need to do so to ensure successful weight loss.*

Unrefined coconut oil can work well as a flavor enhancer in coffee (instead of a sweetener) if you enjoy the taste of coconut; it is also a good way to have more of this healthy oil in your diet.

Alcohol

Here's some good news for those of you who enjoy consuming alcohol in moderation. Alcohol needn't be completely off the menu even when your goal is to lose weight. So long as we avoid the excessively high carbohydrate and sugary "junk" alcoholic drinks, a serving or two a day of the right kind of alcoholic beverages is fine.

Remember that overindulgence and binges, even on the relatively low carbohydrate choices below, could set you back on your weight loss goals. If binges are a regular thing, losing weight will become far more challenging than it need be. As with most good things, moderation really does rule when it comes to alcohol.

Approved Alcoholic Drinks—Yes, There Are Such Things!

From a health and weight loss perspective, we suggest that you limit yourself to one or two servings of alcoholic drinks per day. With that said, here is our list of approved alcoholic drinks:

Red wine—very low in carbohydrates—around 1 gram per serving

Dry white wine—still low in carbohydrates—around 2 grams per serving

Whisky/scotch—virtually zero carbohydrates

Brandy/cognac—virtually zero carbohydrates

White rum—virtually zero carbohydrates

Gin—virtually zero carbohydrates

Tequila—virtually zero carbohydrates

Vodka—virtually zero carbohydrates

True low carbohydrate beer/ultralight beer—essentially what you are looking for is a beer that comes in with around 2.5–3.5 grams of carbohydrates per 12 ounces or 350 ml. Be careful, though; not all beers advertised as "light" are low in carbohydrates. By the way, regular beer comes in at 9–15 grams of carbohydrates per serving, and many so-called "light" beers come in at 7–12 grams (that's four times more carbohydrates than the true low carbohydrate beers). To be truly low carbohydrate, a beer definitely needs to have fewer than 7 grams of carbohydrates a serving. For our purposes, we need to consume beers that come in at that 2.5–3.5 grams per serving sweet spot—a good example of this is Michelob Ultra (2.6 grams carbohydrates—not Michelob Light, which has 11.7 grams carbohydrates). Other choices include Bud Select, Labatt Sterling, Michelob Ultra Amber, Miller Lite, and San Miguel Light.

Mixers For Spirits

When it comes to a choice of mixer for the spirits mentioned above, it is important to avoid fruit juices and obviously sugary soft drinks like cola, lemonade, and "energy" drinks. The best bet is to stick to water, club soda, or a seltzer. If you feel the need for some extra flavor, you can always add a twist of fresh lemon, lime, or orange.

ONE WEEK'S EXAMPLE MENU PLAN

Saturday:

Find and dispose of everything that you will not need in your future. Bag it up and take it to a good cause.
Remember to check your freezer.
Prepare your list of ingredients and bits that you will need to purchase.

╃

Sunday breakfast:
Fried eggs, bacon, tomatoes, and mushrooms

Sunday lunch:
Steak with your favorite healthy vegetables

Sunday dinner:
Portobello mushrooms stuffed with sausage meat, and creamed spinach on the side

╃

Monday breakfast:
Fresh fruit with a little cream

Monday lunch:
Two avocados with plenty of prawns or similar and olive oil

Monday dinner:
Two breasts of chicken, fried or grilled, with melted cheese on top, zucchini/courgettes, broccoli, and string or runner beans

╃

Tuesday breakfast:
Sausages, tomatoes, and plenty of mushrooms cooked in butter

Tuesday lunch:
Tuna and mayonnaise with two avocados

Tuesday dinner:
Baked cod with cauliflower and cheese

ଓ

Wednesday breakfast:
Fresh fruit salad with a little cream

Wednesday lunch:
Omelette with salad and tomatoes in olive oil and oregano on the side

Wednesday dinner:
Steak of your choice with steamed vegetables

ଓ

Thursday breakfast:
A selection of cold meats (salami, etc.) with cheeses

Thursday lunch:
Pickled herrings with beetroot and yoghurt with celery sticks

Thursday dinner:
Prawn and salmon lettuce rolls with a selection of fresh vegetables of your choice

ଓ

Friday breakfast:
Fresh fruit with yoghurt

Friday lunch:
Grilled tuna steak with asparagus

Friday dinner — treat meal:
Jacket potato royal with your favorite cheese, grated
(having a potato is an acceptable treat occasionally; if your
goal is weight loss, don't overdo it!)

CS

Saturday breakfast:
Scrambled eggs with mushrooms on the side

Saturday lunch:
Minced beef in tomato sauce and broccoli

Saturday dinner:
Roast beef with oven-baked vegetables

CS

This example menu is designed to give some idea of the
types of foods you can prepare and consume for healthy
eating. Have a look at the recipe chapter in our original
book, *The ONE Diet* for more ideas. There are hundreds of
cooking combinations you could create. Visit our Web site
to share with others your newfound interest in healthy,
tasty eating.

Cereal Grains

In their natural state, grains, which are the seed head in plants such as wheat, are not digestible by humans. What agricultural man learned to do is to mill the grain, making it somewhat more digestible to us.

However, in doing this, the fibrous element of grain is largely removed—so when we consume flour (and products containing flour); we are eating a processed and refined source of carbohydrate that is of poor nutritional value.

As a side note, a similar occurrence happens with fruit juices, because the fiber has largely been removed from the fruit in the pressing/juicing process, what we are left with is an almost pure sugar drink.

Grains are really quite inedible; have you ever tried eating grains straight from the head of a wheat plant? As we have noted, for humans they need to be milled or ground and then cooked just to make them palatable and digestible by the human gastrointestinal (GI) tract.

Another key issue with cereal grains is that they contain several antinutrients, including protease inhibitors, phytates, alkylresorcinols, and lectins. Lectins, for example have the effect of decreasing the intestinal absorption of many nutrients that are beneficial to us. In addition, what calcium there is in whole grain cereals is blocked from absorption by the phytates.

Wheat also contains gluten, which is a prolamine peptide and is indicated in many diseases now affecting the Western world, such as type 1 diabetes, celiac disease, multiple sclerosis, and rheumatoid arthritis.

When consumed in large amounts, as is typical in the modern Western diet, grains wreak havoc with most people's metabolism and health. As research scientist Loren Cordain notes, *"Many of the world's people suffer disease and dysfunction directly attributable to the consumption of these foods."*

Our society has seen a large increase in calories consumed, notably since the 1970s, and these calories have largely come from carbohydrates derived from grains and sugar. The prevalence of grains and sugars in the typical Western diet is unprecedented in our evolutionary history and is one of the major causes of excess fat, obesity, diabetes, and many more health ailments that affect our population.

Wheat is Just Bad News

White flour and products made from white flour are plain and simply bad news for the human metabolism. White flour has had most of its nutrients processed out of it, leaving nothing but refined carbohydrates.

Whole grain and whole grain products are still no better for us due to their greater antinutrient content, which stimulates intestinal distress and, over the longer term, can cause mineral deficiencies and other health issues.

Potatoes, Starchy Root Vegetables and Rice

We have made the point that starch-rich vegetables and rice need to be limited and for some people avoided, during the process of losing weight. In the case of starchy vegetables such as potatoes, you may find a small portion added to a meal has little negative effect on your weight loss progress.

Grains and grain products are simply best avoided from a weight loss and from a health perspective. The one exception to this rule is white rice, a nongluten grain that contains far fewer anti-nutrients and less fiber (grain fiber can feed and promote excess bacteria in the colon) than other grains. White rice and products made from rice (e.g. natural rice cakes) may be consumed occasionally when the portion size is reasonable so long as you don't observe any negative effect on your weight loss progress.

Once you have attained your goal weight or size, you can fully reintroduce starchy vegetables and white rice into your daily diet, carefully noticing any effects they have on your weight/size.

Is Dairy Healthy For Me?

Dairy products seem to be fine for some people and not so beneficial for others, and it largely comes down to the natural sugar contained in milk, called lactose, and additionally the dairy protein, casein. Those who are lactose intolerant obviously need to avoid milk.

Ghee, butter, and full-fat cheese contain no lactose, and full-fat cream contains only a very small amount. All of these options are likely to be fine even for those who are lactose intolerant.

Half-and-half or half cream, Jersey/Guernsey "Gold Top" milk, and regular whole (full-fat) milk contain lactose in sufficient quantities that they need to be avoided by those who are lactose intolerant. The rest of us can experiment to see how these products affect us, and if we enjoy consuming them. We recommend that they are used minimally—e.g., in recipes, or added occasionally to hot drinks rather than consumed as a drink by themselves, particularly whilst on a weight reduction diet.

Milk and cream that have not been pasteurized or only minimally pasteurized are better for us than brands that are labeled as homogenized, filtered, ultrafiltered, microfiltered, and ultrapasteurized or ultra-heat treated.

The closer the product is to nature, the better it is for us.

Milk, has been marketed to the public as being a good source of calcium. Calcium however, is often better absorbed from other sources, such as broccoli, leafy greens, salmon, and sardines.

Goat dairy can be a suitable alternative to cow's milk, if you enjoy the taste, as it contains less lactose and less casein — in fact, it is more similar to the nutritional profile of human breast milk.

The Reasons to Avoid Low-Fat Milk and Low-Fat Dairy Products

There is a greater percentage of sugar in terms of the sugar to protein/fat ratio in reduced-fat dairy products, which is not helpful for us in terms of weight loss.

Additionally, when the fat content in dairy products has been reduced, the number of fat-soluble vitamins, particularly vitamins A and D, is also reduced. Without the fat-soluble vitamins found naturally in milk and dairy, our bodies struggle to effectively utilize the protein and minerals contained in dairy products.

The Polyunsaturated Fats: Omega-6 and Omega-3

The most common polyunsaturated fats in the human diet are omega-6 and omega-3.

Typically, in Western, affluent countries, we consume far more omega-6 (largely from vegetable, grain, and seed oils) than omega-3 (found in foods like oily fish and meat from cattle raised on pasture).

Ideally, our consumption of omega-3 to omega-6 needs to be at a 1:1 ratio, but in westernized countries, this ratio can be out of balance by as much as 1:50! The problem with an imbalance favoring omega-6 is that it can thicken the blood and increase the risk of chronic diseases, including cardiovascular disease, and the potential risk for heart attack.

Omega-3, conversely, helps to thin the blood, reduce inflammation, and aids in the long-term repair of the body. The take-home lesson is simple: we need to reduce our consumption of omega-6-containing oils. This effectively means completely eliminating vegetable, grain, seed oils and products that contain them (with the exceptions of the previously mentioned unrefined virgin coconut oil which consists primarily of saturated fats and virgin or extra virgin olive oil, which is an acceptable oil rich in monounsaturated fat that we can use for dressing salads).

In other words we need to avoid oils such as sunflower, corn, soybean, safflower, canola, peanut, flaxseed, and products that contain them, which include most processed foods, mass-marketed mayonnaise, salad dressings, and fried foods (except those you fried in butter, ghee, or coconut oil).

Omega-3 oils, as mentioned, occur naturally in oily fish and meat.

With oily fish, there is a health concern due to the toxins they may contain because of the pollution levels in our oceans. The best types of fish with the typically lowest amount of toxins include salmon, tuna, anchovies, Atlantic herring, cod, Atlantic mackerel, sardines and trout.

With regards to cooking oily fish, it is necessary to cook slowly and gently, avoiding high heat; this will help preserve the healthy oils in the fish as much as possible.

Fact: Organic and pastured eggs also contain DHA (docosahexaenoic acid)/omega-3.

The benefits of a balanced intake of omega-3 and omega-6 fats include improved heart health, a healthy fatty acid balance within our cells, improved brain health and function, and improved protein synthesis after exercise.

In addition to this, omega-3 has been shown to be beneficial in reducing prostate tumor growth and increasing survival rates. There are also links with reduced risk of breast cancer.

Simply by eliminating vegetable, grain, and seed oils from your current diet and consuming meat, pastured or organic eggs, and occasionally (once or twice a week) oily fish, too, your omega-3 to omega-6 ratio will be in a healthy balance.

Chocolate Lover?

What many people mean when they say "I like chocolate" is actually "I like sugar and milk solids with a hint of chocolate flavor." Natural chocolate is an acceptable treat. When we are talking chocolate, we mean real dark chocolate, which is around 85 percent cocoa solids.

Dark chocolate makes for a reasonable treat in moderation for those who enjoy the taste of real chocolate. If you are used to eating milk chocolate, we grant you, this is going to take some getting used to. However, over a period of several weeks, as your taste buds adapt to less sugar in your diet, some of you will begin to enjoy the rich taste of quality dark chocolate as an occasional treat.

Low-Calorie Artificial Sweeteners

It is common and understandable thinking to believe that by using low-calorie artificial sweeteners in place of sugars, we are doing a good thing for our weight loss goals.

This is the reason that many people looking to reduce their weight can be seen sipping on diet sodas or adding artificial sweeteners to their beverages, believing that because these sweeteners have zero or very low calorie counts, they will aid their fat loss progress.

There are a couple of issues with this. Firstly, many artificial sweeteners are unnatural chemical compounds that the human metabolism is not used to processing. Some of the artificial sweeteners on the market may even have long-term health ramifications.

Secondly, by continuing to consume sugar replacements, we are keeping our taste buds in training to desire unnaturally sweet foods. This ensures our addictive craving for refined carbohydrates and sugars remains, making long-term weight loss more challenging than it need be.

Artificial sweeteners may trick the mind and body into expecting and priming themselves to deal with high-calorie simple carbohydrates. In reality, they are getting the zero-calorie replacement, and this can actually stimulate our hunger for more food, as the body has not got what it was expecting.

How Many Meals a Day?

It is worth bearing in mind that many of us are used to consuming some form of energy every couple of hours, or even more often. The body does not require this; in fact, most of us feel hungry and eat again whilst our body is still processing what we last ate.

The fitness, health, and nutrition industries have often made a point over the last couple of decades of telling us to eat a little and often, with up to six small meals a day. Our opinion is that this is unnecessary in terms of both weight loss and general health. The notion that humans have to eat in this way for optimal health and weight loss goals is unfounded. In fact, if we had to eat like this, it is doubtful that our species would have ever survived.

We are not necessarily suggesting that you only eat twice a day (although that is a strategy that works very well for some people). The point is not to get caught up in the notion that you have to eat a particular number of times a day, or, for that matter, at set times during the day.

You could eat twice a day or three times a day and healthily lose weight—so long as you are eating the right types of food. Find what works best for you. Relax if scheduling means you have to skip an occasional meal- in fact this may do you some good, as we'll explain when we talk about intermittent fasting.

The Best Quality Meat and Animal Products

Ideally, see if you can source meat that has been pastured (fed grass) or finished on pasture, as opposed to grains. Just as humans have not evolved to eat large quantities of grain, the same is true of most animals. The fat contained in meat sourced from animals fed grain is higher in omega-6 fatty acid—the type we already get far too much of in the West.

This is yet another example of how modern agriculture has altered the food that ends up on our plates. The growing trend of increased awareness amongst health-conscious Americans about this situation has led to an increase in popularity of pastured and pasture-finished meat being labeled as such. In the United States, seek this meat out as best you can.

In the United Kingdom and Europe, the awareness of this situation is somewhat lower and our European readers will perhaps find it more challenging to find meat labeled as pastured. The closest to a solution for our European readers, and what we recommend, is to buy organic meat whenever you can afford to do so. Often the packaging will state what the animal has been fed, and hopefully at least part of its food consumption will have been provided from pasture.

Which Animal Products Are Most Important to Purchase Pastured?

1. Eggs. Buy pastured or organic eggs whenever possible, as the quality of the fat in eggs is greatly determined by the diet of the parent animal.

2. Poultry, pork, and other nonruminant meat. Buy pastured or organic whenever possible, as the quality of the fat in the meat of these animals has a strong correlation with the quality of diet fed to the animal.

3. Fish is another good source of animal protein and fat. When you can, buy wild fish sourced from deep, unpolluted waters. Organic farmed fish are a next-best choice, but avoid regular farmed fish when possible.

4. Beef, lamb, goat, and meat from other ruminant animals contain perhaps the healthiest animal fats that humans consume. The fat contained in ruminant meat that has been pasture fed or pasture finished/organic will be of excellent quality. However, even standard grain-fed ruminant meat will be healthier for us than the first three categories in this list, and so meat from ruminant animals is the least critical to purchase pastured/organic if you are on a budget or have trouble sourcing pastured meat.

Nuts or Not!

Many people are fine eating raw nuts. However, there are some individuals whose digestive systems may find it a challenge to digest nuts. This is due to elements of the nut that can cause indigestion in some people. If you find this to be the case for you, you can simply avoid nuts, or follow the procedure below to make the nuts more digestible.

Firstly, you will need to soak the raw nuts in salt water overnight. Then take the nuts out of the salt water and rinse them thoroughly. Next, ensure they are dried properly (to avoid mould forming); the quickest way to do this is to put them in the oven on the lowest heat possible until dried.

Facts About Fiber

In addition to the natural sugars contained in plants, cellulose is found in their rigid cell walls. Cellulose is a fiber, which humans are unable to digest. The right amount of fiber in our diet helps with the smooth functioning of our gastrointestinal tract.

Optimally, any fiber in our diets will be derived from vegetables and fruits (as is the case when you follow The ONE Diet) and *not* from the fiber in grains.

When you are following The ONE Diet, you will automatically be getting an appropriate amount of fiber in your diet, primarily from vegetables and secondarily from the fruits you eat.

Despite what many of us have been told in the past about the benefits of fiber, too much dietary fiber (especially fiber derived from grains) actually has a negative effect on our health, as it may enable excess bacteria to flourish in the colon, which can cause discomfort, gas, and even irritable bowel syndrome.

Dealing with the Aftermath of Grain and Sugar Addiction

Putting excess grains and sugars into the human system is a lot like putting very low grade/impure fuel into a car. Yes, the car will go, but it won't work optimally or efficiently, and, over the long term, the engine will get clogged, with the impurities in the fuel putting unnecessary stress on the mechanism, leading to an early breakdown.

The car would have run more smoothly, more efficiently, and have had a longer working lifespan had decent fuel been used in the first place.

As it is for the car, it is for the body—put in higher quality food and the body will respond by working more efficiently and effectively, potentially lasting longer. Moreover, in terms of the human body, this means improved general health, less body fat and literally more miles per gallon.

When you drastically reduce your consumption of grains, sugars, and the products that contain them, you will quite possibly feel withdrawal symptoms. It works something like this: You get a twinge of hunger and your mind will go to a chocolate bar, a slice of pizza, or bread. To someone new to eating more healthily, this craving may become very strong—the comfort foods of the past are coming back to haunt. The initial positive buzz of refined carbohydrate energy is being remembered.

STOP...what your body is actually telling you is that it needs food. It might need a lot or it might just need a little. Nevertheless, it needs an input of energy fairly soon. It doesn't even need this energy immediately, but your body is reminding you that it will need some food soon.

So take the time to think about what you are going to eat next; do you have it to hand, is it at home or do you need to go shopping to pick it up?

Just thinking through these thoughts will often abate the immediate hunger. You've shown your mind that you have noted your body's needs and will address them soon or at the appropriate time.

If you still feel a little hungry after finishing your meal, we suggest it is best for you to wait ten to twenty minutes or so. Often it takes that amount of time for the food to "land" and your body to tell your mind that it now has been fed, so all is well, and those hunger receptors can be turned off.

I've followed the nutritional plan for four weeks and I'm hardly losing any weight. What specifically do I need to do next?

You are likely one of a very small percentage of individuals whose metabolism is currently particularly sensitive to food intake. Follow the steps on this and the next page, work your way down the list until you begin to see your weight reduce.

1. Ensure you have completely eliminated from your diet all sugars and foods/drinks containing added sugars and sweeteners, all grains and products made from grains, all vegetable oils, margarines, etc.

2. Consume only one or two portions of berries per day as your total fruit intake.

3. Ensure you have minimized your consumption of; starchy root vegetables (such as potatoes, sweet potatoes, yams, parsnips and cassava), rice and milk. If you have done this already and you are not losing weight, eliminate them completely for now.

4. Experiment with intermittent fasting (see next page).

5. Remember, this five-point plan is to kick-start your metabolism. Once your weight is starting to drop consistently, you can experiment with reintroducing some acceptable carbohydrates like starchy vegetables and more fruits back into your diet, observing the effect this has on your weight loss. If you continue to lose one or two pounds of weight per week or your body measurements are decreasing, you are eating the right amount for you.

Intermittent Fasting—The Simplest Guide

Intermittent fasting can boost weight loss results for those at a sticking point. Intermittent fasting simply means going for a little longer between meals than you usually would. Intermittent fasting has been shown to effectively decrease blood pressure, reduce oxidative damage to DNA, lipids, and protein, and improve insulin sensitivity and glucose uptake.

Four slightly differing approaches to intermittent fasting:

—Simply skip breakfast altogether.

—Every now and then, we can just randomly decide to skip any one of our regular planned meals during a day.

—We may deliberately limit ourselves to just two planned meals on a particular day—one in the morning and one in the afternoon or evening—and no eating on that day outside of the two meals.

—We can have a pre-planned fast for eighteen hours straight through.

When intermittent fasting, avoid overeating in the periods before or after the fast; the aim is to eat what you need, not more to make up for what you haven't had or won't be having over the coming hours.

Changing the Eating Habits of a Lifetime

Imagine that you have learned to type with two fingers. You have mastered typing fast with your two index fingers, but one day you discover that other people can type much faster than you can. You realize that you too could type faster if you changed your way of typing.

It appears that with two fingers you may reach a speed of sixty words a minute. However, with all your fingers you could double that speed. Initially you may be eager to switch typing styles and experience a feeling of excitement when you think about it.

Here we reach a dichotomy. In order to develop a faster typing style, we will need to stop using two fingers and start using all of them. The difficulty arises when we realize that our typing has now slowed down considerably. Where you were typing sixty words per minute, now you are down to twenty-five words a minute. The temptation is to switch back to typing as you have in the past. Correct persistence is required if you are to successfully make the transition.

The temptation to go back to using two fingers is compelling. There could be frustration and anger developing. There could be embarrassment that you have to slow down and that others in the office will see that you are fumbling with the keyboard and making several errors.

Concentration will need to be developed in order to speed up. You will, in a matter of days, notice that your speed is improving and that you are almost up to your old speed, and day by day you are increasing that speed.

Then the day arrives that you break your previous record and exceed sixty words a minute. Each day there is an improvement until you reach your full potential. Suddenly you realize that two things have occurred. The first is that you are typing faster than you have ever typed in the past. The second is that you no longer need to focus on your typing technique the whole process has become automated.

With the help of this book, we anticipate that initially there may be some resistance to changing your dietary consideration. The probability is that your existing patterns will seek to be satisfied and will fight for continuity, on the basis that it is what our mind has become accustomed to and what it knows. However, just as in the typing example above, with correct persistence you will be able to win at weight loss.

Chapter 10.

Boost Your Body with the Best Exercise

"When diet and exercise are properly understood...gone will be the days of weighing food, counting calories, and plodding along on the treadmill for hours. When you eat a proper diet, and partake of high-intensity exercise, you set into motion a vicious positive cycle that makes the body you desire easy to achieve." Doug McGuff, MD

The Role of Exercise in Fat Loss

The role of exercise in fat loss is often overstated, yet it is important when done correctly. The biggest misunderstanding made by many people is the belief that low or medium intensity exercise such as "aerobics" or "cardiovascular exercise" can burn off plenty of calories.

Although it is beyond the scope of this book to discuss the subject of exercise in its entirety, it is worth our while to cover the fundamentals of exercise as it relates to weight loss and well-being. For those who wish to understand exercise fully, we highly recommend reading *Body by Science*, written by Doug McGuff, MD, and John Little.

There is one form of exercise that easily wins when it comes to improving metabolism, building healthy lean tissue, and driving our bodies to "burn" off stored fat. The form of exercise we are talking of is high intensity strength training. When applied correctly, high intensity strength training need be performed only once or twice a week for a maximum of twenty minutes per session.

The Effects of High Intensity Strength Training on Weight Loss and Hunger

High intensity strength training has a unique effect on our bodies when it comes to losing weight that no other form of exercise or activity can match. When we perform a high intensity strength training workout, we kick into action a cascade of beneficial metabolic effects.

Initially there is a release of adrenaline, which then requires the body to utilize large amounts of glycogen (stored energy) out of our muscles. This has the effect of emptying our muscles of their excess glucose, which will need to be replaced.

To do this, our bodies will restore the insulin receptors on the muscle surface; levels of glucose in our blood stream then drop. Following this hormone-sensitive lipase begins to enable the release of our own stored body fat to use as an immediate energy source. This is what actually happens when you "burn" off fat.

There is another huge benefit to the fact that your body is now using its own supplies of stored fat to create energy, and that is, hunger levels actually decrease.

When you eat and exercise in the way we recommend, you will be burning off your body fat and your hunger levels will decrease. When you do feel hungry, it will be noticeable as a subtle signal to think about getting some food soon, rather than, "Oh my goodness, I've got to have something sugary right now!"

You will notice that when you follow our advice, even when you do feel that gentle sensation of hunger, if you ignore it for five or ten minutes it will fade, and you won't notice it again for a while.

Plus, you will only feel hungry when your body cannot get enough energy from using its own fat stores for its immediate needs. In this scenario, your body is essentially burning off its own fat stores as fast as it possibly and healthily can.

By combining our healthy, natural diet with a once- or twice-a-week, twenty-minute, high intensity strengthening program, you are giving your body the metabolic advantage that is your birthright and you will be maximizing your personal genetic potential to look, feel, and be the best that you can, no matter what your current size or age.

High intensity strength training creates a further benefit for our weight loss goals and that is our muscles will be able to store more glycogen. This means even if we do occasionally eat too much, less of that food energy will be converted into fat as our muscles will be able to store more of the glucose as glycogen.

High intensity strength training also increases levels of the hormone adiponectin. Adiponectin can help to combat major health issues, including coronary artery and cerebral artery disease and fattening of the liver, and simultaneously improves both insulin sensitivity and triglyceride (fat) metabolism.

"Resistance exercise does increase REE (resting energy expenditure) and adiponectin in an intensity-dependent manner.... It appears that resistance exercise may represent an effective approach for weight management and metabolic control."

You'll notice that this research published in *Diabetes Care* in 2009, also mentions that high intensity strength training increases resting energy expenditure, which is another massive bonus for those of us looking to reduce our weight.

What this means is that after you've finished your twenty-minute workout, your body is consuming elevated amounts of energy. So long as you're not overeating the wrong types of food, you'll have stimulated the body to "burn" off its own fat even when you're resting or just carrying out your normal daily activities, long after the workout has finished.

This particular piece of research showed that resting energy expenditure remained elevated for forty-eight hours after the workout. This is even before your body has synthesized new lean tissue (muscle) as a result of the workout, which will then lead to an even greater fat-burning effect over the rest of the week till your next workout. Now that really is a great return on investment for your twenty minutes spent working out once or twice a week.

Resistance exercise also increases lipolysis (fat burning) during and after the workout by stimulating the release of the hormones epinephrine, norepinephrine, and growth hormone. One study showed that fat oxidation was 105 percent higher after resistance training than in the control group.

The Core Benefits of High Intensity Strength Training

- Burns calories and turns our bodies into more efficient fat-burning machines by raising our metabolic rate

- Helps normalize body fat levels and improves our physical appearance—the sexy, lean, and toned look

- Improves health issues, including blood pressure, diabetes, heart disease, and cholesterol levels

- Improves heart function and cardiovascular condition

- Strengthens and "tones" the muscles

- Increases our physical energy levels

- Protects our joints

- Improves our ability to perform most other physical activities

Your High Intensity Workout

We recommend that everybody start out with a workout known as the "Big Five," as suggested by Doug McGuff, MD, and John Little in *Body by Science*, which consists of the following exercises performed on good quality weight machines:

1) Seated row
2) Chest press
3) Pulldown
4) Overhead press
5) Leg press

These five exercises efficiently and effectively work all the major muscles of the body including the postural muscles like the abdominals.

You will perform all the exercises in a smooth and controlled manner. This means performing the exercises slowly, not rushing through the movements. Your speed of movement will be around five seconds up and five seconds down, or slower. This deliberate speed of movement eliminates momentum from the exercises, ensuring that your muscles do all the work.

The aim is to do each exercise until the targeted musculature is fatigued and you can no longer move the resistance. Find a weight for each exercise in your initial workout that allows you to perform the movement for between forty-five seconds and two minutes. For example, on your first workout, you may manage to get these times with an appropriate weight for you on each exercise:

> Seated row—ninety-five seconds seconds
> Chest press—eighty-eight seconds
> Pulldown—ninety seconds
> Overhead press—seventy-three seconds
> Leg press—ninety-eight seconds

You are only to perform one single "set" of each exercise that ideally lasts somewhere between forty-five seconds and two minutes.

Use a stopwatch to record your times for each exercise and note them down immediately—this way, you can track your progress from workout to workout. Even a couple of seconds' increase in each movement from one session to the next shows improvement in your body. Once you can perform an exercise at a given weight for longer than two minutes that is a sign to increase the weight used on that exercise at your next scheduled workout.

You may take a brief rest break between each exercise of up to a minute, but once you've started an exercise, continue that particular exercise until physically you cannot perform another repetition with good technique. Do not stop for a rest, then start the same exercise again—once you have started the stopwatch, you keep going on that exercise until you can do no more; stop the stopwatch, record your time, then move onto the next movement.

You will be performing this workout once or twice a week, leaving a minimum of four days between workouts. So if you perform your first workout on a Monday the earliest you will perform your next workout is Friday—or you could just wait until the following Monday.

The recovery time between workouts is where your body will actually be making the positive changes the workout has stimulated, so it is important that you leave at least four days between workouts. Working out more frequently will ultimately stymie your progress.

To learn more about this type of exercise and to view technique videos of each exercise and complete workouts visit Dr. McGuff's Web site, www.bodybyscience.net. You can find a personal trainer or gym in your area that specializes in high intensity training, by going to the Directory page on that Web site.

An alternative for those who don't have access to decent exercise equipment or a trainer is the ebook *Hillfit: Strength* by Chris Highcock available at www.hillfit.com. This short book teaches the reader how to apply high intensity training principles safely at home, without any special equipment.

Are You Sure I Don't Need to Do More Exercise?

Please bear in mind that excess exercise can halt weight loss progress. Remember that using low or medium intensity exercise to burn off calories is extremely inefficient (it takes a heck of a lot of activity to burn off a relatively small number of calories), and too much exercise stimulates unnecessary hunger.

Many people fall into the trap of believing that because they exercised for an hour, they can treat themselves to a sweet "treat." An hour on the treadmill may cause 250 calories more to be metabolized than if you were at rest. At the same time, a well-known regular, individual-size chocolate, nougat, and caramel bar contains 280 calories. So even before you take into account the massive 42.6 grams of carbohydrate in the supersweet chocolate bar, if you run for an hour on the treadmill, then eat one of these bars, you've already consumed more calories than you used by running on the treadmill.

We also need to consider the fact that low or medium intensity activity (e.g., jogging, running, aerobics, etc.) carried out for durations like our example of the hour on the treadmill will likely result in a loss of muscle tissue over time due to overuse atrophy. It's usually quite a slow process, but over the course of a year, a person could lose around four pounds of muscle tissue from this type of training.

Loss of muscle tissue, of course, means a lowered metabolic rate, which means the body burns or uses fewer calories twenty-four hours a day. This will lead to more fat storage—it's that vicious cycle again! Keep this important point in mind: a person who believes exercise can make up for poor dietary habits and excessive carbohydrate consumption is fighting a losing battle.

You've now been introduced to an exercise method that will maximally stimulate fat loss and optimize metabolically important lean tissue, a method that you can perform in just twenty minutes once or twice a week. Do you need to do anything else?

The short answer is no! You will have covered all the health and weight loss benefits that can be derived from exercise in your high intensity strength training sessions. You will have achieved all those benefits in an efficient, effective, and safe manner.

There is no need to spend hours per week at the gym, in an aerobics class, pounding the streets running, on the treadmill, elliptical trainer, vibrating machine, indoor rower, or any other type of equipment. In fact, doing too much medium intensity exercise can not only slow or even halt your weight loss progress but it also puts your joints under too much repetitive strain that may lead to long-term health issues.

What we do highly recommend in addition to high intensity strength training is *recreation*. What we mean by recreation is physical activities you engage in for sheer pleasure.

Walking or, Even Better, Strolling

We are big fans of walking. Just getting outside for a stroll or even a hike when you have the time gets your body moving in a very gentle and natural way. It will also enable you to get some fresh air and some very beneficial sunshine (think vitamin D production).

We're not talking about speed walking or anything like that; we're talking about strolling, ambling along, enjoying the sights and sounds, taking some time for yourself to recharge your batteries and to get the blood gently flowing.

If you can get outside for a daily walk of between ten minutes and an hour, or several short walks throughout the day/evening, we guarantee you'll feel good. We recommend that everyone take at least a short walk every day.

The Benefits of Daily Walking

- Improves your immune system

- Improves mood

- Improves quality of life

- Improves sense of well-being

- Relieves stress

- Increases blood and oxygen flow throughout the body, including the brain

- Provides an opportunity to reflect and ruminate

- Is low impact on your joints

Sports

Some people may enjoy participating in a recreational sport, anything from squash or tennis to an informal game of football in the park. So long as *you* enjoy it and don't overdo it, or push yourself too hard or too often, it will add benefit to your life. Remember, these are not activities you have to do. Only get involved in a sport if you enjoy it and it is pleasurable for you.

A Word of Caution

For some people, when they begin to make lifestyle changes, they can go over the top and think if some exercise is good, then more must be better. Those people may spend a lot of money on an expensive piece of exercise equipment or gym membership that they use for a couple of weeks and then forget about. Or, they may become obsessed by exercise and drive themselves to over exercise nearly every day until they burn out.

Remember, healthy lifestyle choices add to your life rather than take away from it, giving you more energy on balance rather than depleting your reserves. Exercise is similar to food, in that too much of it is ultimately as bad for us as too little. Avoid running your body into the ground through obsessively over exercising.

Perhaps you'd enjoy dancing as a recreational activity. Joining a local salsa class or any other style of dancing can be a lot of fun, plus you'll have some personal interaction — and for those of you who are single, you may even meet someone you'd enjoy dating!

Of course, there are other possibilities for recreation, too, and they don't need to be overly physical. Many people derive benefit from a weekly or monthly massage or learning to relax and switch off through meditation.

Explore these and other options to find which recreational activities work best to enhance your life.

Chapter 11.

Super Successful Strategies

Select one of the strategies suggested below and work through it. Once you feel you have mastered it, you may select another strategy to work on. Avoid trying to do more than one strategy at a time.

Needs and Wants

Whilst conflicts exist between what we need and what we want, there will be a struggle to contain the "fat fight." It is therefore important to create an atmosphere of understanding, cooperation, and tolerance for both if we are to accomplish our objectives.

This strategy requires that we acknowledge the current state of our needs and our wants. It requires that we step out of our emotions and take the stance similar to that of a relationship counselor.

We simply stand between the two elements "without taking either side" and just explore what the current views are from both our needs and wants as if they are two separate parts of ourselves.

By treating needs and wants as if they are two separate entities, we are more able to understand each part's viewpoint better. It is only when we understand the driving force behind our actions that we can be in a place to seek and find a better solution that satisfies our needs and wants.

The key to this strategy is simple: do not take either side. It is not about who is right and who is wrong; it is about understanding each side's position and showing compassion with each. It is about befriending both needs and wants. It is about being able to be a good friend to both if we are to avoid a yo-yo relationship where each side has thoughtless control and abuses the other.

The Strategy

Make approximately thirty minutes available without being disturbed (no phones, TV, etc.) and find a comfortable chair. Perhaps sit with a pad and pen nearby in case you need to make notes, and imagine to your right and left each part preparing their position to present to you.

Internally communicate with each part separately and give enough time for each to tell you their story. In some cases, it may sound like history where the story is mostly about what they had missed out on. In some instances it may be, that you will be informed of how they had been denied sweets through their life, or that they were treated badly and that this is a kind of payback for those years.

Make notes where you need to. Get as true and meaningful an understanding of the drivers behind the behaviors of both your "needs" and "wants." Be caring and sincere about their respective perspectives.

Remember, it is not about who is right and who is wrong; it is more about hearing what their conflict is about. It may be that "needs" has the expectation of being super fit with the stunningly toned body of a sixteen-year-old cheerleader.

Okay, so that is what is desired and sought. The likelihood of that happening we know to be unrealistic, but just hear what their perspective is and how they have reasoned it out.

There is no right or wrong; there just "is." It is just the state of affairs, and this is a report of the state of the union between "needs and wants." Think about each perspective and review the information received. Understand that there may be many truths and that they exist within you.

By following this process, we are finally getting to grips with the victims in this tragedy. Both "needs" and "wants" have a right to what they perceive as being their prerogative and drive. The erroneous thoughts, once brought to light, will impact on our understanding and therefore our future action.

It is anticipated that by understanding the drivers, a change in direction will ensue. Keep in mind that it may be that the original expectations were unrealistic. It may be that both "needs and wants" will learn about each other and respect each other's perspective. It is highly likely that the newfound information contained within this book will have changed your perspective in any event.

Consensus is where we seek a point of agreement, unlike compromise, where both parties in a negotiation have to give up something. When we realize we are in the midst of a futile war, where no progress can be made and the only thing that happens is the destruction of our resources, we can begin to see that carrying on is futile.

Perhaps each part may realize that the other is struggling and that at the end there will be two losers and ultimately you all lose. If that is where consensus is, then great progress has been made. Disease and discomfort will be the final outcome if we continue doing what we have always done.

By allowing expression of needs and wants, we might discover reasons for maintaining our size and shape that we had not previously acknowledged. The drivers that motivated this perspective may result in a new perspective being developed that includes needs and wants working in harmony.

Have a go and discover what needs to happen for you to be at peace with your size and weight.

Self-Awareness

As mentioned previously, we need to be aware of what we look like in order to realize what we need to do to correct the situation. In some instances, we might be shocked at realizing the situation is worse than we have imagined.

This strategy will help bring about new motivation where needed or calm the mind where it had become overly desperate. It requires that a clear and accurate picture of your body shape and size is represented to your mind anew.

The image we hold of ourselves tends to be a snapshot of that we have attached to, which rarely gets challenged. It may be that we have seen an image of ourselves in a picture or a video and stuck with it.

This can be evidenced when we meet up with friends who we have not seen in years and are surprised at how much they have changed. Only then do we stop and have another look at how we have aged and "grown."

It is as though a new perspective was hoisted upon us and woke us up to a realization that we were previously oblivious to. We do age and we do change shape. Often we need this type of jolt to get into action.

We may see an old friend and discover that we had not realized just how much they consumed at a dinner. It may be that we are the ones that seem to go crazy at the restaurant, ordering enough for three. Our awareness may bring us to the realization that in fact we overconsume in comparison to someone who is able to maintain a healthier body than ours.

The Strategy

Make the necessary time available to ensure that you are able to bring about the actions required. Using a digital camera (often found on mobile phones), in your private space, start to take pictures of yourself from as many angles as possible.

Start with full body shots from front and back. A timer may be appropriate to take the photograph, unless you have a partner who is helping to facilitate your change program. Take shots of side views, back views, standing, sitting, slouching, etc., and, once collected, inspect the perspectives as an observer. Avoid becoming emotionally involved.

Now have a look at each photograph. Does it fit in with what you thought you looked like? Is it better, is it worse or is it as you thought? Now just consider, with the knowledge you have, what has caused your body to become as you see it. Is it lack of awareness, is it denial, is it lack of information, is it lack of realization? Explore and sense what seems to be the case for you. It could be a combination of things.

Next, decide if you want to do anything about this. If so, decide what you can do with the resources you have. Start small and be consistent. It is pointless becoming desperate about the situation. This will only instill fear and result in more anxiety being created, thereby defeating the object.

Select a plan from the suggestions in this book and quietly get on with what needs to happen to get you to the place where, when you take the time to look at yourself properly again, you can see a difference occurring. Avoid seeking perfection, as you will discover; unless you are suffering from narcissism, there is no such thing as perfection or imperfection. Therefore, you are evolving into a new you every day.

Let at least a month go by before you start the process again.

Picture the Outcome

In accordance with the way our mind operates, the clearer the outcome we seek, the more likely our mind will "will" us there. Remember that what we dwell upon becomes the focus of our attention. So, it would be prudent to avoid being focused on what we do not want. It makes more sense to have an image of what we do want to look like.

The Strategy

If you have a photograph of yourself looking close to how you want to shape up to be, then have that image on your computer screen or somewhere like the fridge door. Keep the image of the shape you are aspiring to reach foremost in your mind.

In the event that you are unable to find such an image, look in a magazine for a photograph of the shape you seek to be that does not show the facial features of the person in the photograph. It is an image of the shape you seek, no more than that.

Keep in mind that your mind is not stupid, and having an image of a person that is not your body type will do nothing but aggravate the situation. Keeping it real keeps it alive.

Best Friend

Some people may need to have external support. This in many ways is why so many join groups and organizations that specialize in weight control. There are compelling reasons in being with a group.

There is a camaraderie that develops in a group that would otherwise not exist for a person doing this on his or her own. There is a pressure to please your facilitator. There is also useful information that individuals share in a group that can give fresh ideas and can inspire those who have struggled. It is a great place to be encouraged and celebrated when someone accomplishes a goal.

For some people it is important to have this level of support, and, where possible, we would encourage support for those that feel that they cannot do this on their own. Better to have support than to suffer in silence.

In the event that you cannot cope with the whole group thing, you might find that enlisting the help of a very close and supportive friend brings you just what you need in terms of support—a little like having a sponsor, who will be there at times when you just need to let off some steam.

Remember, this will be a short dependence, as we would estimate that within a month or two, you will have completely changed your eating habits. You might find that you accomplish more with having someone to talk to.

The Strategy

Enlist the help of someone who you consider dependable and nonjudgmental. Explain the task that you have set yourself and that you will need supporting for a short time. This will involve the person committing to be there for you in an emergency and agreeing that you will contact him or her once per week with your progress.

Explain that it will not involve him or her giving you any nutritional information and that he or she will not have to do anything whatsoever other than talk with you in the event you have the need to let off some steam.

From your part, you will need to commit to calling the person once per week with your progress report, no matter how you are progressing. Good weeks and not-so-good weeks, you still need to call. You have made a contract with someone by enlisting his or her support, so you will need to honor your side of the deal.

In an ideal situation, it would be handy if it were not someone you see every day, though this would not be unmanageable. Someone perhaps who you know and now lives some distance away.

Having the support does not mean that you become unreasonable and call any time of day, no matter how you might be feeling. Respect for others extends respect to you. So be considerate, and should they be unable for whatever reason to continue, just accept that it is in your best interest and ensure that closure is appropriate.

Criticism and Self-Image

All criticism converts to become self-criticism. When you are comparing other people's size detrimentally, you are then focused on the negative aspects of weight loss. Remind yourself that what you focus on and what you allow yourself to dwell upon is what your mind perceives you as being and wanting.

If the objective is to make yourself feel better by observing another person's misfortune, you are going about it in the most destructive way possible. You will either become the object of ridicule/comparison, or you will live in the fear of being the same as the very person you are being critical of.

It is really simple: just accept that everyone is doing the best he or she knows to do. Not making a judgment simply requires that you can observe, yet have no opinion about him or her. Others are simply humans being. Accept that you may not know what caused that person to be as they are and just move on.

When it comes to self-criticism, you will need to be vigilant. The mind is a "yes" mechanism. Whatever we say to ourselves is met with a "yes" response. If you say, "I am so fat," the mind acts by accepting this literally. If you were to say, "This is difficult," your mind responds with a "yes" and then ensures that it makes it so.

Have no doubt of the importance of the words you are using about yourself and when you speak of yourself and others. The mind does not differentiate between saying things about others and saying things about ourselves. What matters, and can often be evident in the intimation of your tonality, is your intention.

Let's explore what happens when something negative is said. If you were to say, "She's a fat cow," the mind seeks to extract meaning. What is your point? So what? Which means what?

If what you mean is that she is "in some way ugly," then it is likely that you also, on some level and at certain times, look at yourself in some way as being ugly, or at the very least worry that you might be seen as "fat and ugly."

In essence, it is all about projection. Whatever you say of others is simply a projection of yourself. You are talking about yourself through another. The key is to be aware of such negative statements.

Be conscious of your intention. Is it that if you can see someone else as being worse than you are, that makes you feel temporarily better? If it is so, then you will need to understand that this type of thinking leads to self-deception and makes the process of weight loss for you fraught with dangers.

The Strategy

Keep your thoughts "good." You know when you are being good; there is a kindness about you. You are not judging anyone; you are simply allowing others to be.

If you have nothing nice to say about another human being, then say or think nothing. Just observe, accept, and move on. The less attention you give to where you do not want to be going, the quicker you get to where you want to be.

Initially, you might discover that you have been involved unknowingly in serious self-sabotage through negative projections. Each time you notice yourself saying something negative about another person, correct the situation by finding three positive things to say about them.

Let's suppose that you see someone who is not the size you want to be, and you make a negative statement about her: "She is stuffing her face like a pig, so gross." The implication of disgust is somewhat obvious. Correct this immediately by finding or imagining three positive things about her.

This could be "She has a great eye for color," "She looks after her hair," and "She is very polite to people around her." Should your mind start again, then you will need to find yet another three things. Your mind will soon learn who the boss is. Stamp your authority; show your mind what will happen from now on.

The outcome over a relatively short period will be a calmness that you notice only when you stop to notice how much more at peace your mind is without the constant critic.

Self-Care Development

Self-care is not something that comes naturally to us. It does happen when parents have taken the time and the right approach to instill values that include self-care. Here we are not talking about the "remember to brush your teeth" hygiene care; we are talking about a self-care that includes the care of our body above and beyond hygiene.

Think about the amount of time we spend on shopping for clothing, computers, the Internet, telephones, gossip and newsmongering, bijou items, makeup, our children's and pets' welfare, the time we spend in gyms and solariums and with the infernal television and the like.

The community face we project and maintain, as well as keeping up with the neighborhood appearance, is mostly about care of perceived image and things that make us into someone we want the world to see us as being.

What goes on internally and the comfort level of our body may not get a look in. It is almost as if we do not really matter. We are just coasting along in a state of indifference about our well-being.

Is it not pitiful that we have simply not been taught to care about our well-being on a nutritional level? Is it not strange that in schools we are not taught to think about how to maintain our being? We are not taught how to consume healthy foods that enhance and improve the quality of our own physical, mental, and emotional experience.

The Strategy

Set aside about five minutes per day for approximately a month. Select an area of your nutritional or physical life and explore if you are being as aware and as caring as you need to be. For example, you might start by noting what vegetables are in season. Perhaps do some research and discover what vegetables are grown locally. You might seek out where a local farm is located.

On a different day, you might spend some time considering different muscles in your body, and just ponder on what you can do to make life more comfortable for them. Better nutrition, some movements that might help them develop more strength for you.

Stop, think, and act in your body's best interest.

Common Sense

It is obvious that if you go out shopping without knowing what you want, you are opening yourself up to the probability of being influenced by whatever is around you. You will be at the mercy of the clever advertising, as well as being influenced by the smell of the bakery department and the ready-to-take-home meals.

Common sense implies that we are thoughtful, logical, have considered many aspects of any given situation, and have selected the best solution by considering the consequences of our choice.

It is therefore prudent to think through your actions when considering your nutrition. If you put yourself at risk, you are likely to increase the possibility of compromising yourself.

There are several ways of minimizing the risks, and here we list a few of the most obvious.

Avoid Food Shopping When Hungry

Hunger pangs are a very powerful driver. All we can see suddenly becomes a taste to desire. Often, reasoning is lost as instinct overrides all rational thoughts.

List Your Needs and Wants for the Week

By following a process that you have created yourself, you are far less likely to be persuaded by others to buy something you did not set out to purchase. Lists seriously minimize the chances of being distracted. A key to it is to work out the cost of your shopping on the first occasion and take enough cash to cover the cost.

Lists make it clear as to what is permissible and what is not. They are a reminder of your intention and serve to keep you on track. Use a simple phrase such as *"If it's not on the list, it doesn't exist."*

Use Online Shopping

When possible, shop online if you find there is less temptation for you to pick up unhealthy items. Never subscribe to food sites that will bombard you with their daily offers. Resist being the hamster in the cage that will be subjected to other people's will.

Avoid Free Tasters

Avoid "taste this, it's free" type of offers. There is a reason behind any company wanting you to taste its product. It wants you to buy it. Stop, think, and act in your best interest.

Avoid Free Money-Back Offers

"If you do not like it, we will give you your money back." By tasting it, you open your mind to the possibility of reasoning a way of justifying the purchase. Avoid the temptation.

Only Store What You Eat for the Week

Never keep food in your home that you know to be damaging your system. Stop the "it's just in case someone pops round" or "sometimes the kids bring their friends." Any excuse is just that, an excuse to slip back. If you have anything in your home that is nutritionally damaging, then remember it's a risk.

Avoid Judging Others

It can be just as damaging to sit in judgment of others'
habits, as it is to scold yourself for minor misdemeanors.
The less time spent dwelling on negative elements, the
better. Focus on the goodness around.

Resist Temptation

Become the best carer you can be to yourself. Others may
not fully understand what you have to do to get yourself
healthy. Learn to say "thank you…no."

Use Positive Humor

Humor can successfully disrupt negative and unwanted
emotions. It is by far more beneficial to laugh at the tactics
used by the corporations than to get angry. If you find
yourself attaching to an advert, stop and look at it from an
aspect that allows you to have a laugh. When you are
caught out by some sales advertising, stop, observe, and
think, "How desperate those people are."

Avoid Arguments

There is no mileage in getting into an argument with those around you that persist in maintaining their old patterns. The trap that they are in no longer serves you, and, therefore, engaging in argument—"I am right—you are wrong"—simply keeps you unnecessarily connected to the negative elements of your food intake. Be pleased that others have something that works for them.

Avoid Processed Foods

Now that you have the facts about food that has been tampered with, as best you can avoid purchasing processed foods. Occasionally it may be unavoidable. Let that be the exception, and accept that in the main you can avoid it.

Use Rituals to Your Benefit

Often, for many, having a ritual can have a very beneficial effect. Set time aside to engage in a process that focuses your attention upon an act. Rituals help us to expand our awareness of a subject matter and encourage an interest in a specific topic.

If you create a ritual, such as when shopping you only buy what is on the list, you will, over a short period, learn to be more thoughtful and consequently more selective about your purchases. Another type of ritual is to spend a few minutes every morning, perhaps when you are in the bathroom, planning your nutritional intake for the day.

The benefit of showing your mind what and when you will eat seriously helps to avoid fears that would otherwise be present around food.

Make Contempt Your Stop Sign

Contempt serves as a stop sign in the mind. What we show contempt towards; we are highlighting our disinterest about. This is more for items and things that we would otherwise have bought. We might see a "cat and mouse" ice cream that we would have otherwise been enticed by. Now we show contempt toward it. These items have been partially responsible for the extra fat we are carrying.

If you are uncertain about contempt, study someone who is good at it. Differentiate between being cynical and being contemptuous. The cynic is getting off on it; the contemptuous is disgusted by it.

Never Jest About Your Size

Never, ever joke about your size. Remember that more often than not, your mind cannot tell the difference. Self-made comments such as "Guys like big girls" or "Big is beautiful" may not be in your best interest—not unless you want your mind to give you more of the same. In some ways, you are inviting a dangerous possibility.

The Past is No Longer the Present

Avoid conversations about what you used to do. Talk more about what are you doing now and how you are doing it. Talk about what you have accomplished and how much better things are now that you have developed your style of weight loss. Re-imprinting the past can be dangerous and in most cases needs to be avoided. Stay focused on your accomplishments, even if they appear small at times.

Chapter 12.

In Conclusion

Changes in perception of food, nutrition, and diet are essential to bringing about physical and psychological transformation for our well-being.

The ONE Diet covers the affects of advertising, marketing, and ploys used by the food and diet industries to directly or indirectly, covertly or overtly, breach our defense mechanism so as to render us incapable of tending to our nutritional needs healthily.

With the explosion of television advertising, video, billboards, social media groups, and affiliate programs, more and more opportunities have been created to exploit and control us. We are mostly unaware of the vulnerable position we have been left in.

The quality of our food has been eroded. In many cases the "food" we eat has been modified in such ways that it is damaging to our organism. Most mass-produced foods have been processed to the degree of bearing little resemblance to healthy, natural produce.

Furthermore, the ingredients that dominate the typical modern Western diet are both the cheapest to produce and the most damaging to our health. This includes cereal grains, sugars and sweeteners, plant oils and hydrogenated fats.

The crux of the problem of obesity and weight gain in today's world lies in the dramatic increase in the consumption of refined carbohydrates.

The misconceptions surrounding healthy as to opposed to unhealthy fats is clarified as we understand that all hydrogenated oils and most vegetable and plant oils are unhealthy and can severely damage the system. Conversely, eating natural saturated fats present in real foods is vital and fundamental to human existence.

The mind's ability to continue doing what it has always done, once it has been programmed to do so, is both genius and sometimes a dance with the devil. Our ability to create repetitive programs can leave us trapped in habits that are damaging to our very existence. Unless we stop and challenge the basis for our eating regimes, we will remain trapped in old behaviors.

Psychological considerations have been explored to give insight as to how events in our childhood can severely impact our self-image and beliefs about our abilities. Breaking patterns is the challenge that this book offers. Reviewing self-image and beliefs about who we are and what our life is about needs to come to the forefront of our daily activities for a while.

All the research behind The ONE Diet has been thoroughly explored for those who have a need to get to the truth. The information, in a clear and digestible format, evidences the facts for the discerning reader. In essence, we are now aware that what we had been told in the past about nutrition was a carefully crafted illusion, and the facts speak for themselves.

Just as you would not go to a magician to lose weight, we would not expect anyone with half a brain to think that by taking a miracle pill we are going to alter our nutritional needs. The facts speak for themselves, and there are no alternatives and no exceptions to eating well. Just eat natural foods that have not been tampered with from the lists provided, and the rest is a walk in the park.

Setting realistic goals is vital to developing a healthy body, as is developing a respectful attitude towards yourself and others who are in a similar place. Remember that where you focus your attention is where you are heading.

Sitting in judgment of others has been proven to be damaging to oneself. If you cannot be nice to others or to yourself, then have no opinion. Just get on with what you are doing and treat it as a process. At best, you can teach your mind great things by seeing yourself and others in a better light.

Learning to be kind and considerate will further enhance your experience of living.

Simply use The ONE Diet and the included exercises to achieve your desired weight. Resources are included to make the transition more manageable. The use of a food diary and selected strategies all go some way to helping make the process accomplishable and therefore will more likely to lead to success.

We wish you the very best and would love to hear of your successes on our Web site, **www.theonediet.com**.

Resources

Visit—www.theonediet.com for weekly blogs, free downloads, success stories, recipes, and the latest information.

Follow us on Twitter—www.twitter.com/theonediet

Join us on Facebook—www.facebook.com/theonediet

Change Directions—Georges Philips' companion book, especially for those planning positive life changes. **Visit**—www.change-directions.com

Authors' Web Sites
Georges Philips—www.georgesphilips.com
Simon Shawcross—www.simonshawcross.com

Other Web Sites of Interest
M. Doug McGuff, MD—www.bodybyscience.net
Jimmy Moore—www.thelivinlowcarbshow.com
Chris Highcock's Hillfit—www.hillfit.com
The International Network of Cholesterol Sceptics—www.thincs.org

Recommended Reading

Body by Science —Doug McGuff, MD, and John R. Little
Change Directions: Perceive It. Believe It. Achieve It. —
Georges Philips
Stress Management for Professionals: An Introduction —
Georges Philips and Simon Shawcross
Good Calories, Bad Calories/The Diet Delusion —Gary
Taubes
Hillfit: Strength —Chris Highcock
Influence: The Psychology of Persuasion —Robert Cialdini
My Little Book of Verbal Antidotes —Georges Philips and
Tony Jennings
My Little Book of Mediation — Georges Philips and Tony
Jennings
Stop Thinking, Start Living: Discover Lifelong Happiness —
Richard Carlson
The Body By Science Question and Answer Book —Doug
McGuff, MD, and John R. Little